Table of Contents

Dr Sebi Diet; Is it safe?

The Dr. Sebi diet is restrictive, and it may not include enough important nutrients, which the diet's website does not clearly acknowledge.

If a person adopts this diet, they may benefit from consulting a healthcare professional, who may recommend additional supplements.

Vitamin B-12

Following the Dr. Sebi diet may result in a vitamin B-12 deficiency. A person may be able to prevent this by consuming supplements and fortified foods.

Vitamin B-12 is an essential nutrient necessary for the health of nerve and blood cells and for making DNA.

In general, people following vegan or vegetarian diets and older adults have a risk of B-12 deficiency. Doctors usually recommend that people who do not consume animal products take B-12 supplements.

Symptoms of B-12 deficiency include tiredness, depression, and tingling in the hands and feet. There is also a risk of pernicious anemia, which keeps the body from producing enough healthy red blood cells.

Protein

In the diet, protein helps support the health of the brain, muscles, bones, hormones, and DNA.

According to current guidelines, females aged over 19 should have a daily protein intake of 46 grams (g), while males of the same age should consume 56 g.

Some foods included in the Dr. Sebi diet contain protein. For example, 100 g of hulled hemp seeds contain 31.56 g of protein, while the same amount of walnuts contains 16.67 g of protein. For comparison, 100 g of oven-roasted chicken breast contains 16.79 g of the nutrient.

However, the Dr. Sebi diet restricts other sources of plant protein, such as beans, lentils, and soy. A person would need to eat an unusually large amount of the permitted protein sources to meet daily requirements.

Research suggests that it is important to eat a wide variety of plant foods to absorb enough amino acids, which are building blocks of protein. This may be difficult when following the Dr. Sebi diet.

Omega-3 fatty acids

Omega-3 fatty acids are important components of cell membranes. They support:

brain, heart, and eye health

energy

the immune system

The Dr. Sebi diet includes plant sources of omega-3s, such as hemp seeds and walnuts.

However, the body more readily absorbs these acids from animal sources. A 2019 study indicates that a vegan diet contains little or none of two omega-3 fatty acids, unless the person takes a supplement.

Anyone following the Dr. Sebi diet may benefit from taking an omega-3 supplement.

Recipes

Dr. Sebi's recipes often contain unusual ingredients or his patented botanical supplements. However, a person who is not strictly adhering to the diet could easily adapt some recipes to make healthful, plant-based meals:

Dr. Sebi's 'veggie-ful' smoothie. Try leaving out the date sugar, as the drink may be sweet enough without it.

Zucchini bread pancakes. Maple syrup or coconut sugar could replace the date sugar.

Veggie fajitas tacos. People who consume wheat or corn may prefer these types of tortillas.

Summary

Dr. Sebi diet is a diet program created by the Honduras called him as an intracellular therapist and herbalist. He (Alfredo Bowman) claimed that organic and vegan belonging to the raw food would clean your body cells from toxic and diseases. He founded USHA Healing Village in Honduras to help to teach his ideas of diet and herbal therapy. Though some people have claimed that Dr. Sebi diet has increased their health, but it doesn't offer scientific proofs. You must consult it to your doctor. Is it working? Read this book and solve the myth behind the diet.

What Is Dr Sebi Alkaline Food Diet

Dr. Sebi diet can be combined with alkaline food diet. This has been officially allowed by the herbalist of Dr. Sebi. Natural alkaline of herbal and food diet plants can restore alkali cells of the body to be a homeostasis condition. It is beneficial to cure some diseases when you run or semi-salty food diet. If you get interested in applying this diet, you should eat some certain foods. The diet consists of natural alkali vegetables including nuts, fruits, salt nuts, and vegetables. The foods of alkaline diet can clean body cells, and intracellular to make you healthy and robust. This alkaline diet is based on the diseases that only exist in the acid environment. At balance spot of homeostasis, it makes your body require primary mineral supply to make PH stable.

Dr Sebi Diet Plan for Weight Loss

Dr. Sebi diet is a kind of diet to lose weight. If you want to lose weight, you can apply for this diet program. But, remember, you must follow some real principles of this diet program. Dr. Sebi diet divides some foods into six categories. Those are living hard, dead, hybrid, genetic, and medical classes.

The eating pattern of weight loss program focuses on living and raw foods that are called to be electricity foods. These foods can restore dead body cells and lose weight gradually. You may eat fermented foods including fish, alcohol, iodine foods, meat, and products containing yeast. You should eat fruits, no starchy vegetables, leaves vegetables, nuts, grain, and nut jam.

The sample of daily diet menu is recommended to consist of shake with no almond sugar, pure maple syrup, vanilla, cinnamon, butter, and almond milk. You can eat salad past containing fresh vegetables and almond milk and olive oil sauce for lunch. Mushroom soup and green salad become the right menu for dinner.

What is the Dr. Sebi diet

This diet is based on the African Bio-Mineral Balance theory and was developed by the self-

educated herbalist Alfredo Darrington Bowman —
better known as Dr. Sebi. Despite his name, Dr.
Sebi was not a medical doctor and did not hold a
PhD.

He designed this diet for anyone who wishes to
naturally cure or prevent disease and improve their
overall health without relying on conventional
Western medicine.

According to Dr. Sebi, disease is a result of mucus
build-up in an area of your body. For example, a
build-up of mucus in the lungs is pneumonia, while
excess mucus in the pancreas is diabetes.

He argues that diseases cannot exist in an alkaline
environment and begin to occur when your body
becomes too acidic.

By strictly following his diet and using his
proprietary costly supplements, he promises to
restore your body's natural alkaline state and
detoxify your diseased body.

Originally, Dr. Sebi claimed that this diet could cure conditions like AIDS, sickle cell anemia, leukemia, and lupus. However, after a 1993 lawsuit, he was ordered to discontinue making such claims.

The diet consists of a specific list of approved vegetables, fruits, grains, nuts, seeds, oils, and herbs. As animal products are not permitted, the Dr. Sebi diet is considered a vegan diet.

Sebi claimed that for your body to heal itself, you must follow the diet consistently for the rest of your life. Finally, while many people insist that the program has healed them, no scientific studies support these claims.

How to follow the Dr. Sebi diet

According to Dr. Sebi's nutritional guide, you must follow these key rules:

- Rule 1. You must only eat foods listed in the nutritional guide.

- Rule 2. Drink 1 gallon (3.8 liters) of water every day.

- Rule 3. Take Dr. Sebi's supplements an hour before medications.

- Rule 4. No animal products are permitted.

- Rule 5. No alcohol is allowed.

- Rule 6. Avoid wheat products and only consume the "natural-growing grains" listed in the guide.

- Rule 7. Avoid using a microwave to prevent killing your food.

- Rule 8. Avoid canned or seedless fruits.

There are no specific nutrient guidelines. However, this diet is low in protein, as it prohibits beans, lentils, and animal and soy products. Protein is an important nutrient needed for strong muscles, skin, and joints. Additionally, you're expected to purchase Dr. Sebi's cell food products, which are supplements that promise to cleanse your body and nourish your cells. It's recommended to buy the "all-inclusive" package, which contains 20 different products that are claimed to cleanse and restore your entire body at the fastest rate possible.

Besides this, no specific supplement recommendations are provided. Instead, you're expected to order any supplement that matches your health concerns.

For example, the "Bio Ferro" capsules claim to treat liver issues, cleanse your blood, boost immunity, promote weight loss, aid digestive issues, and increase overall well-being.

Furthermore, the supplements don't contain a complete list of nutrients or their quantities, making it difficult to know whether they will meet your daily needs.

Can it help you lose weight

The diet discourages eating a Western diet, which is high in ultra-processed foods and loaded with salt, sugar, fat, and calories. Instead, it promotes an unprocessed, plant-based diet. Compared with the Western diet, those who follow a plant-based diet tend to have lower rates of obesity and heart disease. A 12-month study in 65 people found that those who followed an unlimited whole-food, low-fat, plant-based diet lost significantly more weight than people who did not follow the diet.

At the 6-month mark, those on the diet had lost an average of 26.6 pounds (12.1 kg), compared with 3.5 pounds (1.6 kg) in the control group.

Furthermore, most foods on this diet are low in calories, except for nuts, seeds, avocados, and oils. Therefore, even if you ate a large volume of approved foods, it's unlikely that it would result in a surplus of calories and lead to weight gain.

However, very-low-calorie diets usually cannot be maintained long term. Most people who follow these diets regain the weight once they resume a normal eating pattern. Since this diet does not specify quantities and portions, it's difficult to say whether it will provide enough calories for sustainable weight loss.

One benefit of the Dr. Sebi diet is its strong emphasis on plant-based foods.

The diet promotes eating a large number of vegetables and fruit, which are high in fiber, vitamins, minerals, and plant compounds.

Diets rich in vegetables and fruit have been associated with reduced inflammation and oxidative stress, as well as protection against many diseases (7Trusted Source, 8Trusted Source).

In a study in 65,226 people, those who ate 7 or more servings of vegetables and fruit per day had a 25% and 31% lower incidence of cancer and heart disease, respectively (9Trusted Source).

Furthermore, most people are not eating enough produce. In a 2017 report, 9.3% and 12.2% of people met the recommendations for vegetables and fruit, respectively (10Trusted Source).

Moreover, the Dr. Sebi diet promotes eating fiber-rich whole grains and healthy fats, such as nuts, seeds, and plant oils. These foods have been linked to a lower risk of heart disease. Finally, diets that limit ultra-processed foods are associated with better overall diet quality.

Downsides of the Dr. Sebi diet

 Keep in mind that there are several drawbacks to this diet.

Highly restrictive

A major downside of Dr. Sebi's diet is that it restricts large groups of food, such as all animal products, wheat, beans, lentils, and many types of vegetables and fruit.

In fact, it's so strict that it only allows specific types of fruit. For example, you're allowed to eat cherry or plum tomatoes but not other varieties like beefsteak or roma tomatoes. Moreover, following such a restrictive diet is not enjoyable and may lead to a negative relationship with food, especially since this diet vilifies foods that are not listed in the nutrition guide (13Trusted Source).

Finally, this diet encourages other negative behaviors, such as using supplements to achieve fullness. Given that supplements are not a major source of calories, this claim further drives unhealthy eating patterns.

Lacks protein and other essential nutrients

The foods listed in Dr. Sebi's nutrition guide can be an excellent source of nutrition. However, none of the permitted foods are good sources of protein, an essential nutrient for skin structure, muscle growth, and the production of enzymes and hormones.

Only walnuts, Brazil nuts, sesame seeds, and hemp seeds are permitted, which aren't great sources of protein. For example, 1/4 cup (25 grams) of walnuts and 3 tbsp (30 grams) of hemp seeds provide 4 grams and 9 grams of protein, respectively (16, 17).

To meet your daily protein needs, you would need to eat extremely large portions of these foods.

Though foods in this diet are high in certain nutrients, such as beta carotene, potassium, and vitamins C and E, they're low in omega-3, iron, calcium, and vitamins D and B12, which are common nutrients of concern for those following a strictly plant-based diet. Dr. Sebi's website states that certain ingredients in his supplements are proprietary and not listed. This is concerning, as it's unclear which nutrients you're getting and how much, making it difficult to know whether you'll meet your daily nutrient needs.

Not based on real science

One of the biggest concerns with Dr. Sebi's diet approach is the lack of scientific evidence to support it. He states that the foods and supplements in his diet control acid production in your body. However, the human body strictly regulates acid-base balance to keep blood pH levels between 7.36 and 7.44, naturally making your body slightly alkaline.

In rare cases, such as ketoacidosis from diabetes, blood pH can go out of this range. This can be fatal without immediate medical attention.

Finally, research has shown that your diet may slightly and temporarily change your urine pH but not blood pH. Therefore, following Dr. Sebi's diet will not make your body more alkaline.

Dr. Sebi's nutrition guide details specific foods allowed on the diet, including:

Fruits: apples, cantaloupe, currants, dates, figs, elderberries, papayas, berries, peaches, soft jelly coconuts, pears, plums, seeded key limes, mangoes, prickly pears, seeded melons, Latin or West Indies soursop, tamarind

Vegetables: avocado, bell peppers, cactus flower, chickpeas, cucumber, dandelion greens, kale, lettuce (except iceberg), mushrooms (except shiitake), okra, olives, sea vegetables, squash, tomatoes (only cherry and plum), zucchini

Grains: fonio, amaranth, Khorasan wheat (kamut), rye, wild rice, spelt, teff, quinoa

Nuts and Seeds: Brazil nuts, hemp seeds, raw sesame seeds, raw tahini butter, walnuts

Oils: avocado oil, coconut oil (uncooked), grapeseed oil, hempseed oil, olive oil (uncooked), sesame oil

Herbal teas: elderberry, chamomile, fennel, tila, burdock, ginger, raspberry

Spices: oregano, basil, cloves, bay leaf, dill, sweet basil, achiote, cayenne, habanero, tarragon, onion powder, sage, pure sea salt, thyme, powdered granulated seaweed, pure agave syrup, date sugar

In addition to tea, you are allowed to drink water.

Plus, you may eat permitted grains in the form of pasta, cereal, bread, or flour. However, any food leavened with yeast or baking powder is banned.

Foods to avoid

Any foods that are not included in the Dr. Sebi nutrition guide are not permitted, such as:

- canned fruit or vegetables
- seedless fruit
- eggs
- dairy
- fish
- red meat
- poultry
- soy products
- processed food, including take-out or restaurant food
- fortified foods
- wheat
- sugar (besides date sugar and agave syrup)
- alcohol
- yeast or foods risen with yeast
- foods made with baking powder

- Furthermore, many vegetables, fruits, grains, nuts, and seeds are banned on the diet.

Only foods listed in the guide may be eaten.

Here is a three-day sample menu on the Dr. Sebi diet.

Day 1

Breakfast: 2 banana-spelt pancakes with agave syrup

Snack: 1 cup (240 ml) of green juice smoothie made with cucumbers, kale, apples, and ginger

Lunch: kale salad with tomatoes, onions, avocado, dandelion greens, and chickpeas with olive oil and basil dressing

Snack: herbal tea with fruit

Dinner: vegetable and wild-rice stir-fry

Day 2

Breakfast: shake made with water, hemp seeds, bananas, and strawberries

Snack: blueberry muffins made with blueberries, pure coconut milk, agave syrup, sea salt, oil, and teff and spelt flour

Lunch: homemade pizza using a spelt-flour crust, Brazil-nut cheese, and your choice of vegetables

Snack: tahini butter on rye bread with sliced red peppers on the side

Dinner: chickpea burger with tomato, onion, and kale on spelt-flour flatbread

Day 3

Breakfast: cooked quinoa with agave syrup, peaches, and pure coconut milk

Snack: chamomile tea, seeded grapes, and sesame seeds

Lunch: spelt-pasta salad with chopped vegetables and an olive oil and key lime dressing

Snack: a smoothie made with mango, banana, and pure coconut milk

Dinner: hearty vegetable soup using mushrooms, red peppers, zucchini, onions, kale, spices, water, and powdered seaweed

The bottom line

The Dr. Sebi diet promotes eating whole, unprocessed, plant-based food.

It may aid weight loss if you do not normally eat this way.

However, it heavily relies on taking the creator's expensive supplements, is very restrictive, lacks certain nutrients, and inaccurately promises to change your body to an alkaline state.

If you're looking to follow a more plant-based eating pattern, many healthy diets are more flexible and sustainable.

Dr Sebi Cookbook and Recipe for Weight Loss

ORGANIC FOODS

For optimal health it is essential that we eat only non-hybridized organically grown produce. Conventional or industrial produce are grown with pesticide, herbicides, synthetic fertilizers, and other chemicals that are toxic and harmful to the body. Organic foods are grown without the use of these harmful substances; therefore they taste better, are nutritious and are less dangerous to our bodies.

During the vast majority of our existence on this planet, what choices did we have for food? What could we have eaten during the first 50,000 years before we discovered fire, tools and implements to kill animals? The original diet of Homo sapiens must have been vegetables, fruits and nuts! What other choices did we have? A raw, plant based diet is the main food staple throughout the vast majority of the history of humankind! Before humans began killing and eating dead animal carcass, they ate fruits, leaves, nuts and berries.

EATING PROPERLY

Are you addicted to food? Many of us have become addicted to certain foods. Most people have about 5 or 6 foods that they are actually addicted to and have trouble releasing. These foods are usually hybrids and include rice, beans, soy, breads, potatoes, potato chips, coffee, teas, sweets, chocolate candy, fish, carrot juice, and due to high content of sugar, many are addicted to cigarettes.

Kamut Raisin Pancakes

- 2 cups of Kamut flour
- 1 cup of maple crystals
- 2 tsp of vanilla extract
- 1 2/3 tsp of seams powder
- 1 1/2 cup of almond milk
- 1/4 cup of raisins

Putting it all Together:

1. Put Kamut flour, seamoss powder in a bowl
2. Add raisins, vanilla extract, and maple crystals
3. Stir in almond lik
4. Pour into heated pan and cook evenly on both sides

Seamoss Breakfast Shake

- 4 bp of almond butter
- 1 cup of maple syrup
- 3 cups of almond milk
- 3 tsp of vanilla extract
- 2 tsp of cinnamon
- 1 tsp of seamoss
- 3-4 cups of water

Putting it all Together

1. Blend hot water and seams
2. Add almond butter, maple syrup, cinnamon, vanilla extract and
3. almond milk
4. Blend until smooth and serve

Spelt Strawberry Waffles

- 2 cups of spelt flour
- 1/2 cup of almond milk
- 1/4 cup of water
- 1 tsp of seams
- 1/4 cup of agave nectar

- 1 tsp of vanilla extract

- 6 strawberries cut into small pieces

Putting it all Together:

1. Put spelt flour, seams, and strawberry pieces

2. Add agave nectar, vanilla extract, water, and almond milk

3. Mix together and pour into waffle maker and cook

Cream of Rye

- 1 1/2 cup of cream of rye

- 1/2 cup of water

- 1/2 cup of almond milk

- 1 tsp of vanilla extract

- 1/4 cup of agave nectar

Putting it all Together:

1. Add water to a pot and bring to boil

2. Once boiling, take opt off the fire

3. Add cream of rye mix until thickens

4. Add vanilla extract, agave nectar and milk

5. Stir then serve

Blueberry Spelt Muffins

- 1/4 tsp of sea salt
- 1/3 cup of maple syrup
- 1 tsp of baking powder 1/2 cup of sea moss
- 1/2 cup of sea moss
- 3/4 cup of spelt flour
- 3/4 cup of kamut flour
- 1 cup of almond milk
- 1 cup of blueberries

Putting it all Together:

1. Preheat oven to 400F.
2. Place baking cups in a muffin pan
3. Combine flour, syrup, salt, baking powder, and seamoss together in a
4. mixing bowl.
5. Add almond milk. Mix
6. Fold in blueberries

7. Pour into baking cups and bake for 25-30 minutes

Spelt French Toast

- 2 slices of Spelt Bread
- 1 cup of Almond Milk
- 2 tsp of Quinoa flakes
- 2 tsp of spelt flour
- 2 tsp of maple crystals
- 1/2 tsp of sea salt

Putting it all Together:

1. Mix all together
2. Dip bread till soak but not soggy.
3. Add olive oil to pan to lightly fry on both sides

Kamut Puff Cereal

- 1/4 cup of agave nectar
- 1 cup of hot Almond milk
- 1/4 of raisins

- 1/4 cup of chopped almonds
- 1/4 cup of chopped dates
- 1 cups of kamut puffs

Putting it all Together:

1. Add almond milk to:
2. Almonds, cereal, dates, agave nectar and Enjoy!

Papaya Breakfast Shake

- 2 cups of almond milk
- 1/2 cup of agave nectar
- 1 tsp of seams
- 1/2 cup of cold water
- 1/2 cup of fresh or frozen papaya

Putting it all Together:

1. Blend water and seamoss
2. Add Papaya, milk, and agave nectar
3. Blend till smooth and serve

Cream of Kamut

- 4 cups of almond milk
- 2 cups of water
- 1 1/2 cup of kamut flour
- 1 1/2 tsp of vanilla extract
- 1 cup of maple crystals
- 1 tsp of cinnamon

Putting it all Together:

1. Make like cream of rye

Pasta Salad

- 2 boxes of spelt penne
- 2 avocados cut in small pieces
- 1 1/2 cup of sun dried tomatoes
- 1/2 cup of chopped onions
- 1/4 cup of almond milk
- 1/4 cup of fresh lime juice
- 3 tbs of maple syrup
- 4 tbs of sea salt

- 3-4 dashes of cilantro
- 1/2 cup of olive oil

Putting it all Together:

2. Cook the pasta as directed on package
3. Add everything in a big bowl
4. toss until evenly distributed

Mushroom Patties

- 2 portabella mushrooms
- 1/2 cup bell peppers
- 1/4 tsp oregano 1 Pinch of cayenne pepper
- 1/4 bunch of cilantro
- 4 tbs sea salt
- 1 tsp dill
- 2 tsp onion powder
- 1/4 cup of spelt flour

Putting it all Together:

1. -Soak mushrooms for 1 minute in spring water

2. -Remove and place in food processor with scallions and bell peppers

3. -Add cilantro, flour and other seasonings

4. -Mix thoroughly and form patties

5. -Place them in heated pan with 2 tbs olive oil

6. -Fry on both sides until done (approximately 3 minutes each)

The Greatest Greens

- 3 bunches of mustard and turnips greens 1/2 of each
- 2 cups of chopped onions
- 1/4 cup olive oil
- 1 tsp of cayenne or chili powder
- 3 tbs sea salt

Putting it all Together:

1. -heat pan then add onions, cook till golden brown

2. -add greens, cook down for 20 min.

3. -season with sea salt, and cayenne or chili powder

Stuffed Bell Peppers

- 1 1/2 cup of quinoa
- 1 lb. oyster or brown button mushroom
- 2 green bell peppers
- 3 tbs olive oil
- 1/2 red bell peppers chopped fine
- 1/4 tsp of ground cumin
- 1/2 tsp sweet basil
- 1/2 tsp dill
- 1/2 tsp sea salt
- 2 slices of kamut or spelt bread toasted, crumbled

Putting it all Together:

1. -steam bell peppers until tender, then hollow out
2. -place quinoa grain in saucepan with water covering the top

3. -cook low heat until water is absorbed, then set aside
4. -sauté mushrooms and red bell peppers in olive oil
5. -season inside bell peppers with some spices and olive oil
6. -mix quinoa, mushrooms, and red bell pepper with remaining
7. seasonings
8. -stuff bell peppers with mixture, then sprinkle bread crumbs on top
9. -bake in preheated oven at 250 degrees for 10-15 minutes
10. -serve hot and enjoy with a green leafy salad

Vegetable Mushroom Soup

- 1 lb oyster mushrooms, chopped
- 1 cup quinoa
- 1 small red and green bell pepper chopped
- 1 bunch spinach, washed, and steamed
- 2 tbs olive oil

- 1/2 lb kamut spiral pasta
- Spring water
- 2 onions chopped finely
- 2 large chayote squash, peeled and chopped
- 2-3 bunches kale
- 1 clove
- 1/2 tsp: marjoram, rosemary, oregano, thyme, red pepper, and cumin

Putting it all Together:

1. -put olive oil in hot skillet
2. -sauté mushrooms, bell peppers, and onions slowly for 20 minutes
3. -add mushroom mixture in soup pot and fill with spring water
4. -add chayote squash
5. -add thyme, marjoram, rosemary, oregano, red pepper, cumin, clove,
6. and quinoa
7. -Simmer 45 minutes
8. -add Kamut Pasta simmer for 15 min

9. -add spinach, stir, and then serve when tender

Vegetable Patties

- 1 bunch of broccoli chopped fine
- 1 bunch of kale greens cut fine
- 2 chayote squash diced
- 1/2 red and green peppers chopped
- 1 medium yellow onion chopped fine
- 1 pinch of African red pepper 3 tbs olive oil
- 1/4 cup seamoss powder
- Spring Water
- Kamut Flour

Putting it all Together;

1. -heat skillet with 3 tbs olive oil
2. -add onion, bell pepper, chayote squash, African red pepper and
3. ground cumin, sauté 2-3 minutes
4. -add broccoli and kale simmer 10-12 minutes
5. Preparation for Kamut flour:

6. -mix seamoss with enough flour and water to make a dough

7. -roll out on floured board cut into 10" diameter circles

8. -place cooked vegetables 1/2 of circle

9. -fold other half to cover the vegetables

10. -use a fork to pinch the edges closed

11. -place patties on lightly greased baking sheet and bake 20-30

12. minutes or until golden brown

Homestyle Okra

- alb fresh okra diced
- 2 soft tomatoes
- 1/2 yellow onion chopped fine
- 1/4 tsp ground cumin
- 4tbs olive oil
- 1/4 tsp African red pepper
- 1/4 tsp. sassafras
- 1/4 tsp. sea salt cooked wild rice or quinoa

Vegetable Stir Fry Medley

- 1 pkg. oyster mushrooms, sliced
- 2 zucchini, sliced
- 1/2 small yellow onion, chopped fine
- 8 cherry tomatoes, chopped
- 3 tbs olive oil
- 1 cup broccoli, chopped fine
- 1 small red and green pepper, chopped

1. Putting it all Together:
2. -Put olive oil in heated stainless steel wok
3. -add tomatoes and onions
4. -add your favorite seasonings and sauté 3-4 min
5. -add mushrooms and sauté another 3-4 min
6. -add zucchini, bell peppers, broccoli and sauté 3-4 minutes

Wild Rice

- Spring water
- 1 medium yellow onion chopped fine

- 1 small red pepper
- 1 cup mushrooms, chopped medium, fine (oyster or brown button)
- 1/8 cup olive oil
- 1 tsp. thyme
- 2 tsp. oregano
- 1 tsp. sea salt
- 1/8 tsp. African red pepper

Putting it all Together:

1. Soak rice in spring water over night for best results
2. -Cook rice according to package instructions and set aside
3. -pour olive oil in hot skillet
4. -Sauté vegetables and mushrooms 2-3 minutes
5. -Add thyme, oregano, sea salt, and African red pepper
6. -Fold in Cooked rice and simmer for 20 minutes

7. Tip: If you forget to soak rice over night:

8. Par boil rice for 20 minutes set aside loosely covered until rice opens

9. (approx. 2-3 hours)

10. Rinse and cook until tender

11. Or:

12. Boil rice, adding additional water and stirring as needed until tender.

Spaghetti Recipe

- Follow directions on the Vita Spelt Pasta box on how to cook the pasta.
- After the pasta is cooked, strain it.
- In a separate pan add 1/2 cup of olive oil
- 2 cups of tomato sauce
- add 4 tbs of sea salt
- 1 1/2 tbs of onion powder
- 2 tbs of cayenne/chili powder
- 3 tbs of maple syrup
- Heat sauce on medium high for 10 minutes
- Stir pasta into sauce

- Let sit for 5 minutes.

Serve and Enjoy!

Lasagna

- 1 red bell pepper, chopped
- 1 yellow onion chopped
- 2 tbs olive oil
- Bay leaf, crumbled
- Spelt lasagna pasta
- 2 lb., mushrooms
- 8 fresh tomatoes
- Almond cheddar cheese
- Oregano, to taste
- Sea salt, to taste

Putting it all Together:

1. Tomato sauce
2. -Heat Skillet and add olive oil
3. -Place onion, bell peppers, oregano, sea salt, and bay leaf in skillet

4. and sauté

5. -Boil tomatoes for 10 minutes

6. -Place in ice water for five minutes, drain and remove skin from

7. tomatoes

8. -Blend tomato in blender -fresh tomato sauce

9. -Add tomato sauce in skillet with sautéed seasonings

10. -Simmer for 30-45 minutes

11. -Set aside half of sauce to be used to make mushroom sauce,

12. remaining half to be used when layering.

Mushroom sauce

1. -Place mushrooms in water, soak for 1 minute, strain and slice

2. -Season to taste sauté for 2 minutes and add 1/2 of saved sauce

3. (see above), set aside for layering.

Pasta

I. -Prepare pasta according to instructions

II. -Once pasta is done, place under cold water for easy handling

III. -Layer a deep baking dish with tomato sauce

IV. -Place a layer of pasta on top then a layer of mushroom sauce

V. -Then add a layer of almond cheddar

VI. -Repeat steps until dish is almost full

VII. -Place 2 cups of sauce on top of remainder of almond cheddar

VIII. -Bake in 350 degree oven for 20 minutes until almond cheddar is melted

Note: Almond cheddar cheese can be purchased at Trader Joes and Whole Foods Market

Hot Veggie Wrap

- 3 cups diced tomatoes
- 2 cups onion
- 1 cup of diced bell peppers
- 1/2 cup of mushrooms chopped

Putting it all Together:

I. -Stir fry all vegetables for 5 minutes

II. -Warm spelt tortilla

III. -Put together

IV. Enjoy!

Taquitos

- 2 cups of chopped onion
- 4 cups of chopped mushrooms
- 2 tsp chili powder
- 3 tbs sea salt
- 2 tbs tomato sauce
- 2 tbs oregano
- 2 tsp. onion powder
- 2 tsp. ground thyme

Putting it all Together:

I. -Add 1/4 cup of olive oil to the pan

II. -Add onion sauté until golden brown

III. -Add mushroom sauté for 5 minutes

IV.   -Then add seasonings

 V.   -Wrap in corn shells tightly

VI.   -Then fry until crispy

Mushroom Salad

- 1/4 bunch fresh spinach, torn
- 1/4 bunch red leaf lettuce, torn
- 1/4 bunch romaine lettuce, torn
- 1/2 lb. fresh mushrooms
- 1/2 red bell pepper, chopped
- 1 sm. red onion, diced
- 1/2 cup olive oil
- 1/4 cup fresh lime juice
- 1/2 tsp. dill
- 1/2 tsp. basil
- 1/2 tsp. sea salt

Putting it all Together:

  I.   -Thoroughly wash mushrooms, dry, slice

 II.   -Add onion, bell pepper, olive oil, lime juice,
         dill, sea salt, and basil

III.   -Marinade 1/2 hour in refrigerator

IV.   -Thoroughly wash greens, dry and shred

V.   -Place greens with mushrooms and mix thoroughly

VI.   Enjoy!

Vegetable Salad

- 1/2 lb. fresh string beans
- (Remove ends and snap in half)
- 1/2 bunch romaine lettuce, torn
- 1/2 bunch watercress, torn
- 1/2 bunch cilantro, chopped fine
- 1/2 tsp. dill
- 1/4 tsp. cumin
- 1/4 cup fresh lime juice
- 1/2 cup olive oil

Sweet basil to taste

Putting it all Together:

- -Put olive oil in bowl

- -Add dill, cumin, basil, and lime juice
- -Marinade in refrigerator for 1-1/2 hours
- -Mix thoroughly with lettuce, watercress, and cilantro
- Enjoy!

Avocado Dressing

- 3 Ripe avocados, peeled and seeded
- 1/2 small red onion
- 1/2 tomato peeled
- 1/4 cup fresh lime juice
- 4 tbs pure olive oil
- Pinch Cayenne Pepper
- Few sprigs of cilantro
- 1 tsp. chili powder
- 1 tsp. oregano
- 1 tsp. cumin
- 1/2 tsp. sweet basil
- 1/2 tsp. sweet basil
- 1/2 tsp. thyme
- 1/4 tsp. sea salt

Putting it all Together:

I.   Puree avocados in blender

II. Add remaining ingredients and 2 tablespoons
     of spring water

III. Lightly blend and pour over your salad

IV. Note: Season to taste

V.   Use cold pressed, virgin olive oil

Creamy Salad Dressing

- 4 tbs. almond butter
- 2 green onions
- 1/4 tsp. ground cumin
- 1/2 cup fresh lime juice
- 1/2 tsp. sweet basil
- 1/4 tsp. thyme
- 1 tsp. maple syrup
- 1/4 tsp. sea salt

Putting it all Together:

I. In a glass bottle, add all ingredients and 2 tablespoons of spring water

II. Shake thoroughly and enjoy!

Cucumber Dressing

- 3 med. cucumbers, peeled
- 10 almonds, raw, unsalted
- 4 tbs. pure olive oil
- 1/4 cup fresh lime juice
- 1/4 cup green onions, chopped fine
- 1/2 tsp. thyme
- 1/2 tsp. sea salt
- 1/4 tsp. dill
- 1-1/2 cup spring water
- Few sprigs of cilantro, chopped

Putting it all Together:

I. Blend 10 almonds in spring water, 2 minutes, high speed

II. Strain and set liquid aside

III. Puree cucumbers in blender with almonds

IV.   Add olive oil, lime juice and remaining ingredients

V.   Lightly blend, adding liquid, if needed

VI.   Pour over your salad and enjoy!

Xave's Delight

- 2 fresh limes squeezed
- 3 tbs. maple syrup
- 3 oz. sesame tahini
- 1 oz spring water
- 1 tsp. sea salt
- 1/2 tsp. red pepper

Putting it all Together:

I.   In a glass bottle, add juice of 2 limes, water, maple syrup, sea salt,

II.   red pepper, and sesame tahini

III.   Shake well and dress your salad!!

Lime and Olive Oil Dressing

- 1/4 fresh lime, squeezed

- 1/2 cup olive oil
- 1/8 cup spring water
- 1 tbs. maple syrup
- 1/4 tsp. sweet basil
- 1/4 tsp. thyme
- 1/4 tsp. oregano
- 1/4 tsp. ground cumin

Putting it all Together:

- Put all ingredients in a glass bottle
- Shake thoroughly and enjoy this delicious and easy salad dressing!

www.ingramcontent.com/pod-product-compliance
Lightning Source LLC
Chambersburg PA
CBHW031242130726
47988CB00008B/3194